ONE HOUR TO

AMAZING

How to Get in Amazing Shape & Health

in Just One Hour per Week

Dwight D. Miller

Published by Infernal Soul Publishing LLC

Front cover photo taken by Marc Remmen, featuring

Jaclyn Divine and Dwight Miller, at the Lotus Pond

Yoga Studio in Tampa, Florida

Paperback ISBN: 978-0-9984911-0-3

Ebook ISBN: 978-0-9984911-1-0

Also Written by Dwight D. Miller

Dred Wars: Resurgence (an urban fantasy)

This book is for my amazing four children: Tatum, Aubrey, Sydney and Billy; my family; my friends; all the people who ask me how I stay in such great shape, have tons of energy and don't get sick; and for anyone looking to feel better, look better and live a longer, healthier, happier life.

Contents

Disclaimer

The information in this book is for informational purposes only. As each and every individual situation is unique, you should consult a medical professional or health care practitioner, before use or application of the techniques, exercises, diet, health tips, and any other information described in this book. The use or application of the information in this book may have serious health consequences for people with certain health conditions. The use or application of the information in this book may not work for some people with certain health conditions, or for certain body types. Results may vary. The author is not a doctor, scientist, nutritionist, medical or health care professional. The author and publisher specifically disclaim any liability, loss, or risk, personal or otherwise, that is incurred as a consequence, directly or indirectly, from the use or application of the information contained in this book. Please consult a doctor.

Chapter 1

Introduction

There's something about the struggle in life, when you are pushed to your limit, when everything starts to change. You gain new perspectives. Your confidence grows. Your potential expands. You find new meaning in life. And when it comes to your body – when your body is pushed to its limit – your body gains a new perspective. Its one overarching purpose is to keep you alive. So when you push your body to its limit, your body triggers powerful forces within to adapt to this new limit – to heal you, to rejuvenate you, to make you stronger – so that you'll survive it the next time. The good news is that you can trigger these powerfully healthy forces in your body within seconds.

I wrote this book for busy people like me who want to get in shape, look fabulous, feel amazing, and enjoy a healthier life. You can quickly get into amazing shape in just one hour per week – and you'll be including both weightlifting and cardio. I call my workout the "Executive Workout™," because the way it works is quick, efficient and to the point, just like a business executive.

I'm going to show you exactly what you need to do, for just one hour per week, based on the latest scientific studies and my own personal experience. Whether you want to gain muscle, lose fat, or both, the Executive Workout™ is designed to work for you. If you're willing to commit just one hour per week to feel and look better, this book is for you.

People actually stop me when they see me, to ask me how I do it. How do I find the time to stay in shape and look the way I do? How do I have such great energy? How do I not get sick when everyone else gets sick? How am I able to work a more-than-full-time corporate job, raise my daughters, go to their activities, visit my son, spend time with friends – and still find time to write novels? In this book, I tell you how I do it, and why I do what I do. It's natural and simple.

I am forty-six years old. I have three teenage daughters: Tatum (age eighteen) who lives with me full time; and Aubrey (age seventeen) and Sydney (age thirteen), who live with me half time. I also have a six-year old son, Billy, in Florida. I travel there to spend time with him, and I bring him to Arizona in the summer. I am a senior finance manager for a very large public company. My first novel, an urban fantasy entitled *Dred Wars: Resurgence,* was released in September 2016. This book will be released less than four months later.

Right now, and for the past several years, I feel – and have felt – absolutely fantastic, nearly every day. I don't take any medications. I haven't been sick in over seven years, even though at times all of my children have been sick, as well as my coworkers who surround me. I've traveled on several dozen commercial airline flights over this time as well. With some relatively simple changes in what you eat, and a one-hour commitment per week for exercise, I know you can be healthier, feel great and live a better life than you do today. My daughters' health has improved – and so has the health of many others who have followed the philosophies in this book.

Another vital feature that I'm including in this book is the simple eating philosophy that I follow. I tell you what foods to avoid – and which ones are good – and why. If you follow this eating philosophy, you will become a fat-burning inferno, and you will have a lot more energy. I also provide some important information on the most significant health issues in our food supply, here in the U.S., so that you can make more informed choices that will improve your health and the health of your loved ones.

Finally, I'm bringing you a handful of health tips that will give your holistic health a power boost. If you're super busy, and you just want the recipe for getting in shape in one hour per week while staying healthy, I've also provided short summaries of the information, so that you can grab what you need and go.

I want to share something with you. I want to help you. I miss my dad. My wonderful father, Lee Dale Miller, died at the very early age of fifty-eight, due to cancer. We have lost enough loved ones. People are getting sicker, younger. I talk to my friends, my family, my thousands of social media friends, and I look at people whenever I'm out and about. A lot of people have health challenges. I, too, have had struggles over the years, and fortunately, I have had people who helped me through mine. At one time I weighed thirty pounds more than I do today. But what happened to me in 2009, and afterward, changed me forever. This experience warmed my heart – and it made me want to help you.

For me, it was a huge personal and spiritual journey. It really brought to the front of my heart the importance of compassion for others. I'd never had to rely on someone else, and when I found myself injured and suffering, it was truly humbling and heartwarming. I cannot overstate the appreciation I have for those who helped me heal. Now, I ask myself how I can find ways to help others. With this in mind, I hope you find some things in this book that will lead you and your loved ones to a healthier, happier life.

In 2010, two and a half months before my fortieth birthday, around 5 PM on a Saturday, I was rear-ended in my car by a large Chevy Z71 truck. The next day, my legs and lower back were a little stiff, and my left leg felt slightly tingly. When I woke up Monday morning to take my three young daughters to school, my lower back and left leg were in excruciating pain. I couldn't reach down further than my knees. My six-year-old daughter, Sydney, helped me get dressed.

The collision had knocked the bottom disk (L5) in my spine over to the left by one-and-a-half centimeters, placing it on top of my sciatic nerve, right over my sacrum (S1). I was in constant, never-ending pain. You know what it feels like when you hit your "funny bone" – that sensitive spot on your elbow – really hard? It was like that, but much worse. The hot burning, the pins and needles – it just would not stop. That's how I felt from my waist, down my left leg, all the way to my toes. So about one-fourth of my body was radiating pain, twenty-four/seven. Trust me, that's a large area to be hurting. I was also having frequent back spasms, which locked me up in severe pain.

At the end of each day, I would lie on my stomach in bed with a bag of ice on my L5/S1 area. I could not wait for the ensuing numbness. Ice was my new addiction. Every night I had to have her, and she was SO damn good!

What was perhaps even more painful for me, I wondered if my active lifestyle had come to an end. The thought of not being able to play and be active with my little girls broke my heart. Just three weeks before, I had taken my three young daughters, Sydney (age six), Aubrey (age eleven) and Tatum (age twelve), snowboarding in Flagstaff for the first time. It was an incredible memory that I still hold dear, and it was so much fun for us all. I'm looking at one of the pictures of us from that trip – which is on the wall to the right of my computer screen – as I'm writing this. It's shocking how your life can change in an instant.

Just days after the accident, I met with my physician before picking my daughters up from school. After going over the MRI results, the doctor told me that I should see either a pain specialist or a surgeon. I was stunned. My heart dropped through my gut as I felt the sickening emotional shock. Only then did the seriousness of my new predicament hit me. Before this meeting, I didn't know what sciatica was, nor did I understand what was going on inside me.

Sciatica was not an easy thing to fix. Back surgery was a likely option for me, and I've always felt it was a huge gamble. I wasn't excited about the thought of someone sticking a long needle into my spine and injecting me with drugs – or, worse, taking a knife to delicate parts of my spine. Call me crazy.

After the appointment, on the drive from the doctor's office to pick up my little girls from school, I cried all the way, fearing I wouldn't be able to enjoy all of the active things I loved to do. Wrestling with my girls, chasing them at the park, playing sports with them, hiking in Sedona, snow-skiing and snowboarding, rollerblading, working out – everything was at risk now. It was heartbreaking.

Over the next couple of nights, I read everything online that I could find. I discovered that sometimes sciatica could be corrected with physical therapy, so on I went, determined to fix myself without drugs or surgery. But the only thing that the first physical therapist did was what I called "put me on the rack," basically strapping my chest in place on a table, and then using a strong machine to pull straps attached to my ankles to stretch me. The medical people called it traction. All I ever pictured was the racks used to torture prisoners in medieval times. I'm six foot three. I used to joke with everyone that I was five foot eight when they had first put me on the rack.

Also, the first physical therapist instructed me not to be active in any way whatsoever, so when I was at home, I just lay in bed. Since I also worked from home as a realtor, I was now extremely sedentary. Talk about torture for an active person. This wasn't good for my mood either, and my real estate sales and income took a major dive.

I got stretched on the rack five days a week for a while, then four days, and finally three. I wasn't improving, so three months later, the time for a new physical therapist had arrived. The next guy examined me each time we got together and had me do a basic gym workout routine: ride a stationary bike, then use weight machines for the various muscle groups. This did nothing for my sciatica, but I at least felt a lot better physically and mentally, since I was working out a little again.

Six months after the accident, after my second physical therapist had failed to improve my situation, I pondered giving up. It wasn't that they were unqualified: the two physical therapists had a combined fifty to sixty years of experience in physical therapy. Adding insult to injury, during this time I was also going through a divorce. My pregnant wife had left the state with our unborn son. My father was far into a losing battle with stage-four cancer at the young age of fifty-eight. I have never felt as low in my life as I was at that moment.

Looking back at it now, I find that I am deeply thankful for those experiences. The struggles of those dark days absolutely changed my perspective on life, and what I wanted to do with my life. I learned that I'm not the type of person who loses faith easily, that I can take one hell of a beating and will get back up for the next one. It took fourteen months of determination to beat my sciatica. I found a new and profoundly deep spirituality. I discovered what was really important. Money became far less important. More than anything, I wanted to help people.

As I mentioned earlier, people seem to be getting sicker, earlier in life. We are losing loved ones. I see it everywhere around me. The majority of people who are about my age and older do not look healthy. And younger people don't look much better. Moreover, too many people are taking medications every day for some ailment, or to simply feel better.

I have five best friends in life, whom I've known since the age of fourteen or earlier. Four of these friends have children. Two of them have an autistic child. At one point, two of us had girlfriends with autistic children, so four of the five of us were in relationships involving an autistic child. Growing up, I don't remember any autistic children. It floors me to think about how common this condition is today.

Do you see what I see? I know there are a lot of people who, if they made some very simple adjustments, could feel and look so much better naturally, and live lives of much better quality.

Here are some interesting U.S. health statistics:

From the Centers for Disease Control and Prevention (CDC) website on 12/1/2016:

- "More than one-third (36.5%) of U.S. adults have obesity."

- "Obesity-related conditions include heart disease, stroke, type 2 diabetes and certain types of cancer, some of the leading causes of preventable death."

- The estimated annual medical cost of obesity in the U.S. was $147 billion in 2008 U.S. dollars; the medical costs for people who are obese were $1,429 higher per person, per year, than those of normal weight."

- "From 1980 through 2014, the number of Americans with diagnosed diabetes has increased fourfold (from 5.5 million to 22.0 million)."

From the National Cancer Institute's website on 12/1/2016:

- "Approximately 39.6% of men and women will be diagnosed with cancer at some point during their lifetimes (based on 2012 data).

- "National expenditures for cancer care in the United States totaled nearly $125 billion in 2010 and could reach $156 billion in 2020.

I don't want you or your loved ones to be one of these statistics. I want you to live a full, happy and healthy life.

I'm the intellectual sort, being a Gemini, and my strongest intellectual curiosity has always been about the body and about overall health. I started working out when I was fourteen. I took a really challenging nutrition class in college. In college and afterward, I worked out six times a week. Now, when I get time to read articles, I absolutely devour the latest news and research on natural health. It takes time to sort through all of the conflicting information that we get bombarded with. Unfortunately, I think that the health information that comes out of the media is confusing at best, if not downright misleading. You can literally read one article that says one thing – and the next article you read says the opposite. To help sort through this, I've tried to boil down the most significant issues for you in this book.

My goal in this short book is to be efficient, and give you exactly what you need. The Executive Workout™ will help you build muscle and get in cardio shape in just one hour per week. It will unleash powerful healing forces within your body to rejuvenate you and give you more energy. My basic eating philosophy and health tips will help improve your health – and maintain it. It will also boost your energy.

I could say in this book something as simple as "an organic apple is good for you," and there would be people who disagree with me based on some study somewhere, or on their personal philosophies. I wrote this book for all the people I know and love dearly, for those who have asked me how I do what I do, and for those people looking for ideas on how to live a happier, healthier life. The topics in this book are my personal opinion on what has worked for me, and I will often point you to supporting data from doctors and scientists. I encourage you to do your own research, educate yourself and make your own health choices.

I am not a doctor. (I just play doctor in the bedroom sometimes.) I am not a nutritionist or medical professional. I am simply an absolute natural-health nut. I cite a number of scientific studies and quote many doctors, scientists and medical professionals in this book. They are the experts. I sift through the confusing health information that we are bombarded with, much of which is driven by the companies that want you to buy their potentially unhealthy products. I talk to other people who also seem to be exceptionally healthy, and I test what makes sense for me, and for my family.

I think one benefit of me not being a doctor is that you'll actually be able to understand everything in this book. I like to keep it simple, and I wanted to keep this book short. If you want to dive deeper, you can always educate yourself by scouring through the various studies and research, which I greatly encourage.

Before you change your diet, exercise routine, or follow any information in this book, consult a doctor and review your health history. Please, do not skip this step. Your health and well-being are worth at least one doctor consultation. Don't you agree?

Chapter 2

Before you Start an Exercise Program

First of all, consult a physician. Discuss any health issues that you may have, as well as the requirements for your new workout. Once you are cleared to go, here are some important questions you need to ask yourself before you start:

Find Your "Why" and Create a Positive Self-Image

Why Are You Starting This New Program? Maybe you want to lose weight, feel better, improve your health, look better to attract a mate, build muscle, etc. Find the emotional reasons that will really motivate you as you move forward. If you look at yourself in the mirror and don't have any emotional reason to change, you're going to have a hard time accomplishing change.

22

What do you want in life? How do you want to feel? Who is it that you love? Sometimes we just want to get healthy so we will live longer and be there for our loved ones. EMOTION is the key to motivation. Find that feeling, that reason you HAVE to do this – no matter what.

I could not get everything done in my life without an exceptionally strong "why." As you go through this book, you may notice that I like the word "inferno." The name of my publishing company is Infernal Soul Publishing LLC. I envision an inferno inside me, burning brightly – an infinite source of energy, drive and love. I tap into it. I tap into my love of my children. I tap into my love of life. I enjoy feeling fabulous, and I want – more than anything – to help anyone I can to live a happier, healthier life. That's what gets me out of bed an hour or two early to write before I go to work, and keeps me writing until I fall asleep at my desk at night.

Find your why, then create and continue to build a powerfully positive image of yourself. I highly recommend a couple of classic books: *The Power of Positive Thinking* by Dr. Norman Vincent Peale, and *Psycho-Cybernetics: A New Way to Get More Living Out of Life* by Maxwell Maltz, M.D.

Lastly, learn to appreciate all the things you have in life. Too many people focus on what they lack. Before you go to sleep each night, say out loud everything you're thankful for. Life is an amazing gift, and this simple shift to gratitude will have powerful effects on your attitude and well-being.

Where are you starting from?

Though this step is often missed, it is one of the most important ones in your process. It's extremely difficult to improve something that you don't measure. I want you to ask yourself the questions below, then write down your answers on a scale of one to ten:

1. How good have I felt during the last week? The last month? The last year?

2. How much energy do I have on a regular basis?

3. How do I look from a fitness or health standpoint?

4. How much do I weigh?

5. What is my body-fat percentage?

6. What is my muscle mass?

7. How many calories do I burn while resting? (A "bod pod" test will tell you.)

8. What are all my body measurements?

a) Chest

b) Biceps

c) Hips

d) Waist

e) Thighs

Right after I started the weightlifting routine I did a "bod pod" test, which is supposed to be the most accurate way of measuring body-fat percentage and muscle mass, and also calculating the number of calories you burn while resting, which will give you insight about your metabolism. The bod pod encloses you in a pod and measures the displacement of air around you. They used to measure body composition by submerging people in water. Compared to that, the bod pod is a piece of cake, but there may not be many of them near where you live. At many gyms, the staff or trainers will at least have equipment to measure your body fat in some other way. This numerical value is important.

If you are lifting weights, and you're following my guidelines on what to eat and what not to eat, and if all you do is step on a scale to measure your weight – you may get frustrated if you're trying to lose weight and not succeeding. But what could very well be happening is that you're gaining muscle, and that is offsetting your fat loss. If your strength is increasing, that's a really good sign. Actually, though, your body-fat measurement will be a better guide. To be consistent, just make sure that you use the same piece of equipment to measure yourself over time, as different equipment can vary widely. That's why I did the bod pod, because I wanted to have precise results.

What Are Your Goals?

Now that you've established your starting point, where do you want to be when you've reached your goal? By when? You have to write down what your goals are – and make them specific. Really! Write it all down! Even better, write it down with a picture of yourself when you were healthier, or use a picture of that swimsuit model you'd really like to look like. Picture that version of yourself in your goals.

This is important. I want you to be realistic. Time and time again, I've seen people set goals that are too ambitious – even aggressively so – and then they beat themselves up if they don't reach a goal that may have been unreasonable to start with. Then they quit, and moreover, their self-esteem has been damaged.

I want you to set yourself up for success. You – and no one else – define what success is for yourself. Here's an example. Let's say that you've gained forty pounds over the last ten years, and now you want to lose it all. It may be tempting to set a goal to lose all forty pounds in six months. Is it possible? Technically, yes – it's possible. People have lost forty pounds in twenty-six weeks before. To do this, you had better have a life-or-death level of emotional motivation to drive yourself to achieve such a goal. That's over one and a half pounds per week.

But let's say you set a goal of losing half a pound per week. In six months, or twenty-six weeks, that's thirteen pounds. I want you to picture what a pound of meat looks like in the grocery store. Losing thirteen of those is a fantastic accomplishment! Even if it takes a year, that's truly a great accomplishment. For most people, if they are exceeding their goals, it helps keep them motivated. And when you stay motivated, you keep moving forward, and that's all I want you to do. KEEP. MOVING. FORWARD!

If you just keep moving forward, you will start to feel good – people will notice and give you compliments – and you will accelerate toward your goals. EASY button!

Chapter 3

The Executive Workout™, Part One – Weightlifting

This is the shortest, simplest workout that I've ever seen. I named this amazing workout routine the "Executive Workout™" because it is short, to the point and delivers results. A random guy at the gym told me about this philosophy. I researched it online and found that these strength principles have been around for decades. Most of what you read about weightlifting is geared for bodybuilders, or what I call people who are "going caveman." I just don't have the time or desire to try to impress women with my massive biceps anymore. Nor do I think it's healthy to be oversized like that.

I needed a workout that was quick and effective to fit into my busy schedule. When I first tried this particular workout, I was skeptical. But I felt the results immediately. Even though I had been lifting weights regularly for a few months before this new workout, and had lifted for much of my adult life, the results I experienced, and the way I felt, were undeniable and incredible.

I started this new workout in early 2016. At this point I had three teenage daughters, two of whom were in sports, plus a five-year-old son who lived in another state. I also had a more-than-full-time job – and I was writing my first novel, an urban fantasy called *Dred Wars: Resurgence*, and building my author platform. If you're as busy as I was or more, God bless you. So, when I came across this workout, my first thought was,

"OMG! This is too good to be true – but if it actually works, what an incredible way this is, for someone who is so busy with life, to get in fantastic shape and maintain it!"

It is so simple in concept. I can't believe I had never heard of it. When I discussed it with all of my friends, none of them had heard about it either.

Most importantly, I got results, and I got them fast. Two weeks into this workout, I did a bod pod reading to measure my muscle mass and body fat. My body fat was 15.5%. Thirty-seven days (five weeks and two days) later I did a second bod pod reading to measure the change in my body. I am six feet, three inches tall. I'd gone from 172 pounds to 178. I gained six and a half pounds of muscle and lost half a pound of fat. Gaining almost one and a third pounds of muscle per week is not bad for a tall, skinny guy. Think about what a pound of chicken or steak looks like in the grocery store. In just five weeks I was thrilled to take six and a half pounds of muscle and add that throughout my body while losing fat, and I had not done any cardio whatsoever. You would need to consume a lot of protein to build muscle this quickly.

In just five weeks, my shirts were now tight around my arms and my chest. My shorts, jeans and slacks were now tight on my thighs. I literally had to weigh staying on the workout program versus having to buy an entire new wardrobe. When I walked through the corporate office, people stopped to compliment me on how muscular I looked since they had seen me last. I felt fantastic.

Obviously, lifting weights builds muscle. You'll not only look and feel healthier, you'll increase your metabolism – so you'll burn more calories, even when resting. The stress of lifting also makes your bones stronger. I also find that I am very relaxed after a great workout.

To start with, there are just a few primary exercises that you do in one workout, and you can also work on your abs if you want. Although you may be tempted, do not do any more than this, no matter what! Keep it simple.

And, to keep it simple, there are just two different workouts:

<u>Lifting Workout 1</u>:

> Leg Press (use a machine)

> Shoulder/Military Press (use a machine)

Triceps Extensions

Curls

Abs (optional)

Lifting Workout 2:

Bench Press (use a machine)

Lat Pulldowns, Wide Grip (use a machine)

Seated Rows (use a machine)

Curls (optional)

Abs (optional)

It's very important to have good form when you lift weights, so have a trainer teach you good form for each of the exercises in the workout if you don't already know. Do each repetition slowly, counting to at least four or five each time you go up, and each time you go down. This is the absolute key to this workout: go to exhaustion on the last repetition and fight it, fight it, fight it as long as you can, and then go down as slowly as you can. It's all about the last rep. It's all about the struggle. This is why it's best to use a machine. Your muscles will be spent. If you bench pressed with free weights and followed this routine, you would have the weights resting on your chest at the end. Keep good form throughout the struggle so that you don't hurt yourself.

Here is a key point – You only do one set of each exercise. Even though I had been lifting weights for four months before I started this workout, I was sore for three days after doing this workout for the first time. Sore from just one set of each exercise! And the results came immediately. Keeping the muscle engaged continuously for so long, and then pushing it to exhaustion, engages and shreds so much more muscle fiber than the traditional routine. You will feel the difference.

Do just one set of each exercise, taking just two to three minutes of rest between each exercise. For the leg press, you want to find a weight where you can do eight to ten reps. For the other exercises, except for abs, five to seven reps are ideal. Again, fight the last rep as long and as hard as you can. That is the key. As soon as you think you can do the minimum reps at a higher weight, increase the weight at your next workout.

You will literally be in and out of the gym in ten to fifteen minutes. If you feel that this isn't long enough, go and sit in the sauna for twenty to thirty minutes. That'll get you cleansed and relaxed. Drink plenty of water. Eat some whey protein. Do not do additional weightlifting.

When you start this exercise regimen, do Workout 1 and Workout 2 three days apart. You need to ensure that your body gets enough time to heal and build muscle. If you are unable to increase the weight in any given workout from the previous one, first make sure that you've been eating enough and getting enough rest. I cover what to eat in a later chapter. Second, if you're sure you've been eating enough and getting the rest you need, then you need to add another day of rest in between workouts. As your muscles get bigger, they will need more time to heal and rebuild.

For abs, there's no substitute for the "plank". I also enjoy the yoga "boat" pose and "cat" pose. You can do these at home, or at the gym, every two or three days.

I'm a huge believer in building your core to support your back, given that so many people eventually face back problems.

People who exercise often do weightlifting and cardio, but the third category of fitness is often neglected, especially by men. You need to stretch. As you get older, this becomes more and more obvious. There's a basic stretching routine that I've found to be very helpful after the leg press and cardio workouts. I also often stretch when I first roll out of bed in the morning, or any time when I've been sitting too much.

Quick stretch routine:

- First and foremost, always be gentle with yourself when stretching.
- Lie on your back.

- Dip your chin to your chest as you pull one knee to your chest for at least ten seconds while you keep your lower back relaxed. Put that leg down.

- Pull the other knee to your chest for at least ten seconds.

- Pull both knees to your chest while you keep your back relaxed for at least ten seconds.

- Roll onto one side. Pull your heel up against your butt for at least ten seconds.

- Roll onto the other side and repeat.

- Sit up, keep your legs straight and touch your toes. This is the most important stretch if you sit a lot, since spending a lot of time with your legs bent shortens and tightens your hamstrings, which will then pull on your lower back. Keep stretching. Relax your back. Once you reach your toes, then grab your heels from the inside, then grab your heels on the outside of your feet.

How to breathe when you stretch (or any other time of day):

- Always breathe in and out through your nose, if possible.

- Exhale as you're stretching or bending, and exhale completely until you cannot exhale any more air. This clears stale air out of your lungs.

- As you inhale, push your knee or leg in the opposite direction that you were stretching while holding it in place with your hands. For example, if you were pulling your knee to your chest as you exhaled, when you inhale, you hold your knee in place as you push the knee downward as if to straighten your leg. Inhale fully, until you cannot inhale any more air through your nose. As an additional option, you can then breathe in some more air through your mouth, as if you were sipping through a straw. This full breath floods your body with fresh, invigorating oxygen, and it will eventually expand your lung capacity.

- When you begin to exhale again, you reverse back into the stretching motion. You will notice with each exhale that you can usually stretch a little further than the last time.

You'll become aware of the tightness in your legs or back, and you'll soon realize when it's good to stretch throughout the day.

With any new exercise program, you should consult a physician. I am not a doctor. Once again, I would like to emphasize this: High-intensity exercise will put stress on your body. You should get an understanding from a medical professional – given your health history – of the implications that this routine may have for you.

Chapter 4

The Executive Workout™, Part Two – Cardio

Cardio has been my personal nemesis ever since I played high school basketball. Something about running line drills five days a week until I nearly puked cured me of any possible link between running and pleasure. And long-distance running for me is just so dang boring. Thankfully, the same principles that make the Weightlifting portion of the Executive Workout™ effective also apply to this Cardio Workout. In just ten minutes, you can get the same results as a fifty-minute workout. Sound too good to be true?

You may want to consider the research study, published April 26, 2016, in PLOS One: "Twelve Weeks of Sprint Interval Training Improves Indices of

Cardiometabolic Health Similar to Traditional Endurance Training despite a Five-Fold Lower Exercise Volume and Time Commitment," written by Jenna B. Gillen, Brian J. Martin, Martin J. MacInnis, Lauren E. Skelly, Mark A. Tamopolsky, and Martin J. Gibala.

For an easier read, a great write-up of this study was published by The New York Times on April 27, 2016, in the article "1 Minute of All-Out Exercise May Have Benefits of 45 Minutes of Moderate Exertion," by Gretchen Reynolds.

In the most ambitious twelve-week study of its time on interval training, scientists at McMaster University, in Hamilton, Ontario, took twenty-five sedentary men and separated them into three groups:

1. The Control Group – No change in their exercise habits

2. Moderate-Intensity Continuous Training (MICT) – Fifty minutes of cycling composed of:

   a) A two-minute warmup.

   b) Forty-five minutes of continuous moderate exertion

   c) A three-minute cool-down.

3. Sprint Interval Training (SIT) – Ten minutes of cycling composed of:

   a) A two-minute warmup.

   b) A twenty-second all-out sprint (starting at the 2:00 minute mark).

   c) Two minutes of low-intensity cycling.

d) A twenty-second all-out sprint (starting at the 4:20 minute mark).

e) Two minutes of low-intensity cycling.

f) A twenty-second all-out sprint (starting at the 6:40 minute mark).

g) A three-minute cool-down.

Both the exercising groups, MICT and SIT, did one exercise session in the first week, two in the second week and then three sessions per week for the rest of the twelve-week period.

The researchers concluded after this twelve-week study that, "a SIT protocol involving 3 minutes of intense intermittent exercise per week, within a total time commitment of 30 minutes, is as effective as 150 minutes per week of moderate-intensity continuous training for increasing insulin sensitivity, cardiorespiratory fitness and skeletal muscle mitochondrial content in previously inactive men. This investigation represents the longest comparison of SIT and MICT to date and demonstrates the efficacy of brief, intense exercise to improve indices of cardiometabolic health."

In layman's terms, the SIT group showed similar improvements to the MICT group in each area tested in the study, despite only exercising ten minutes per session compared to fifty minutes. Peak oxygen uptake increased 19% in both groups after training.

When I do this routine I simply walk, then sprint in short intervals, around my neighborhood. Usually I can find ten minutes in the morning before work to do this simple routine. If it's winter or raining, you can even do this in a gym around a basketball court. It amazes me how much more energy I have on these days. By 10 AM I am ravenously looking for a hearty snack – just from ten short minutes of exercise – and only one minute of it intense!

Cardio Workout:

Walk for two minutes.

At the two-minute mark, sprint for twenty seconds like a bear is chasing you. Give it everything you've got.

Walk again.

At the 4:20 minute mark, sprint for twenty seconds like there's a tsunami coming up behind you.

Walk again.

At the 6:40 minute mark, sprint like it's a race to all your dreams.

Walk again.

At the ten-minute mark, congratulations! You're done!

The key is to exert yourself all-out for those twenty-second sprints. You should be huffing and puffing for oxygen at the end of each burst. Don't hold back.

So, to really boil this down, this is how I motivate myself to do this routine. Five of the ten minutes is just walking during the warmup and cool-down, and nine of the ten minutes overall is walking. It's really all about the three intense, twenty-second bursts. So I tell myself, "Come on, D, it's only three (insert multiple expletives here) reps of twenty seconds. Anyone can do that. No excuses."

Benefits of High-Intensity Interval Training:

The Executive Workout™ Cardio routine is a type of High-Intensity Interval Training (HIIT). A HIIT routine is simply one where you alternate periods of intense activity with much-less-intense activity.

Here's a quote from the American College of Sports Medicine website (www.acsm.org), in a brochure entitled "High-Intensity Interval Training" (brochure content provided by Len Kravitz, Ph.D.):

"HIIT training has been shown to improve:

- aerobic and anaerobic fitness
- blood pressure
- cardiovascular health

- insulin sensitivity (which helps the exercising muscles more readily use glucose for fuel to make energy)
- cholesterol profiles
- abdominal fat and body weight while maintaining muscle mass"

HIIT engages your fast-twitch and super-fast-twitch muscles versus a traditional steady cardio routine, which predominantly uses slow-twitch muscles. Approximately fifty percent of your muscle fibers are the fast-twitch and super-fast-twitch type. Another huge benefit of HIIT is that it causes your body to produce more human growth hormone (HGH). Production of HGH in your body declines significantly after age thirty. Some of the above benefits for HIIT correlate with the benefits provided by HGH.

Benefits of HGH include:

- Fat burning

- Higher energy levels

- Faster healing

- Boosts your immune system

- Stronger bones

- Lowered blood pressure

Helps rejuvenate your body, including skin and organs, so you look and feel more youthful. The natural decline in HGH may drive your aging process.

After exercising, don't forget to do my favorite stretch routine:

Quick stretch routine:

- Lie on your back.

- Dip your chin to your chest as you pull one knee to your chest for ten seconds while you keep your lower back relaxed. Put that leg down.

- Pull the other knee to your chest for ten seconds.

- Pull both knees to your chest while you keep your back relaxed for ten seconds.

- Roll onto one side. Pull your heel up against your butt for ten seconds.

- Roll onto the other side and repeat.

- Sit up, keep your legs straight and touch your toes. This is the most important stretch if you sit a lot, since spending a lot of time with your legs bent shortens and tightens your hamstrings. Keep stretching. Relax your back.

Once you reach your toes, then grab the heels

of your feet from inside your legs, then outside.

With any new exercise program, you should consult a physician. I am not a doctor. High-intensity exercise will put stress on your body. Sprinting outdoors or around a track, whether on your feet or on a bike, increases your risk of falling and injury. So be careful out there. A stationary bike may be a good idea for some of you. Once again, you should first get an understanding from a medical professional of what implications this routine may have for you, given your own unique health history.

Executive Workout™ Summary

The Executive Workout™ takes just one hour per week, comprised of:

- Two weightlifting sessions of ten to fifteen minutes each ~ thirty minutes per week.

- Three high-intensity interval training sessions of ten minutes each ~ thirty minutes per week.

Chapter 5

What to Eat; What not to Eat

My absolute intellectual passion is reading and learning about food, nutrition and being healthy. As I'm sitting here writing this, I can tell you that I have not had a common cold or virus in over seven years now. My three daughters are in public school and get sick from time to time. All the employees around me get sick at work. I've flown on several dozen commercial flights during the last seven years. All of us are always being exposed to viruses and bacteria. Avoiding the illnesses that they can cause, I truly believe, is all about your immune system being a scorching inferno that zaps anything it comes across.

I and many people I talk to have changed our health and body composition simply by changing what we've chosen to eat. Any bodybuilder will tell you that your eating habits are more important for building muscle than the weightlifting you do.

Part of what to eat depends on what your goals are. If you want to build muscle, you need to eat more protein and more food in general to fuel building more mass. If you want to build muscle and lose fat at the same time, it's a real challenge to find that balance. You need to get enough protein, yet make sure you're not eating too much overall. It's easier to build muscle and then "lean out" (lose fat) afterward, since if you don't eat enough you won't be able to build muscle effectively. Make sense? Plus, building muscle increases your metabolism, so you'll burn more calories and fat even while resting.

A few years ago, one new piece of knowledge and its application totally changed my perception of what to eat. It was a true paradigm shift in my life. Did you know that at any given time, your body uses only one of two sources as its primary source of fuel? You can either burn carbs as your primary fuel, or you can burn fat as your primary fuel.

The overwhelming majority of us burn carbs as our primary fuel. When we eat carbs, our body processes them the same way as we process sugar, namely into glucose. Our body then uses the glucose for energy. How can you tell if your body is running on glucose? Your stores of glucose energy only last for two to three hours. So if you get hungry every two to three hours, that's a sign that you're running on glucose. In the old days, if I didn't eat lunch on time I would get cranky, and sometimes even shaky.

I remember the food pyramid I was taught in grade school that called for eating lots of grains, including bread, cereal, rice and pasta, followed by fruits and vegetables, then dairy, meats/beans/eggs/nuts and finally, fats, oils and sweets. I took a very difficult nutrition class in college when I was working out six times per week. I was very serious about being fit and healthy.

I used to eat a lot of bread, and I still love the taste of it today. I mean come on, not many things smell better than fresh bread in the oven, right? Or cookies? There's nutritious flour grain in every bite. Mmmmm.

Then there's pizza, which my food accolade for was "hot sex in a box." My father owned a Chicago-style pizza restaurant when I was young. Afterwards, I delivered pizzas throughout college and continued devouring it well into adulthood. Pizza was not only cheap but it had lots of grains, vegetables, dairy and meat, so it was basically a superfood straight from heaven, right? It had everything on the food pyramid in the perfect proportions. Well...

Even though I've always been active, with a high metabolism, I put on weight. When my young teenage daughters pulled out an old picture of me at my sister's wedding, they said with excited surprise, "Wow! Dad, you were a fattie!"

Gotta love the brutal honesty of your own children. The truth is, I'm in a shirt and tie in that photo, in a large group of people, so you can only see me from the neck up – and yes, I was much fatter than I am today. I weighed thirty pounds more than I do now. Now, fifteen years later at age forty-six, I weigh the same as I did as a senior basketball player in high school.

Now, my favorite eating philosophy by far is to eat low-carb whole foods. By whole foods, I mean that when you look at it, you can see the natural state of the food because it hasn't been processed. You can see the vegetables, the beans, the rice, the meat, and you can identify what's what.

One low-carb eating philosophy is called a ketogenic diet. A ketogenic diet initiates a process called ketosis, in which your body switches its fuel source from carbs to fat. With this approach, you need to limit carbs to below fifty grams per day, and increase your intake of healthy fats to replace those carb calories. Depending on how much fat you have on your body, you're going to have a much vaster energy supply than the carb-based two to three hours.

There are many benefits of being fat-fueled:

- The first noticeable sign of when you switch to being fat-fueled is that you won't feel cranky or shaky, the way I used to, when you don't eat a meal on time. You won't get cravings for sweets, or food in general, the way you do on a carb-based diet.

- You will become a fat-burning inferno.

- Your blood-sugar and insulin levels won't swing as wildly, so this approach is an attractive option for preventing and dealing with diabetes. If you have diabetes or prediabetes, you absolutely must consult a doctor before changing your diet as it can have severe health consequences.

- You will have great energy.

- You will have increased endurance and stamina.

- Some articles claim that this also reduces blood pressure and improves acne, among other benefits.

Again, it is extremely important to consult a doctor about a change in diet, particularly if you have any health conditions, food allergies or sensitivities. There are definitely impacts to be considered if you're diabetic, have high blood pressure, are breastfeeding or have other health conditions. I am not a doctor. Also, be aware of any food allergies you might have, since, for example, many people have extreme, even life-threatening allergies to foods like nuts or shellfish.

Below, you'll find my list of what to eat and what to avoid in order to shift your body into fat-fueled mode. If you are more hard-core, you can also fast to enter ketosis as you blow far past your reserves of carb energy, which only last two to three hours.

What to Eat and What to Avoid – Basic Health Rules

1. Avoid sugar. Did you know that when they scan your body to detect cancer, they inject you with sugar? Here's a quote from the National Cancer Institute's Nuclear Imaging page at imaging.cancer.gov (Google "cancer test with sugar"): "The radioactive sugar can help in locating a tumor, because cancer cells take up

or absorb sugar more avidly than other tissues in the body." If this is the ONE AND ONLY thing you take away from this book, I will be extremely grateful. Consider this: Whenever you eat sugar, the first thing you feed in your body is cancer cells. When I learned this, it instantly became easy for me to cut out sugar, though I still partake in the occasional sweet treat. My father died of cancer at only fifty-eight. I miss him dearly.

2. Avoid table salt. It has chemicals in it and it can only be bad for you. I've read articles saying that it can be made from heating the water that mixes into crude-oil deposits at high heat, and that it may contain glass and other inedible things. I don't know the full story, but it's probably best to avoid regular table salt.

Instead, use sea salt, and my favorite, Himalayan pink salt, since they are natural and loaded with healthy minerals. (Other naturally occurring salts you might try come from places as varied as England, Sicily and Hawaii, and each has its own distinctive flavor.)

3. Avoid eating chemicals (including pharmaceuticals, unless medically necessary), such as aspartame, hydrogenated oils, preservatives and food coloring. Our body is able to process out some chemicals to a degree, but others build up over time and can begin to interfere with the delicate chemical-based processes that keep our body running smoothly. Have you ever known someone where part of their body stopped functioning normally? Toxic chemical build-up can be a

root cause of this and many other issues. I believe many chemicals are cancer- and disease-causing as well. Look at the ingredients in a loaf of bread at the grocery store. If you make bread at home, it takes only about six ingredients, not the fifteen to twenty you'll see listed in the store's bread. If you're on medications, try seeing a naturopathic physician to see if you can solve your issues naturally, without the prescription drugs and the side effects they cause.

4. Avoid soda. It's loaded with sugar, or high-fructose corn syrup (fructose is a type of sugar), and other chemicals – and the carbonation itself is very acidic. If your diet is acidic, it pulls out alkaline minerals like calcium and magnesium from your body to balance its pH. It's far better

to keep these minerals in your bones, where they're helping to keep them strong. I also believe that a more alkaline diet is important for your energy level. Have you ever noticed that batteries are alkaline? You produce electricity like some amazing type of battery.

5. Avoid beer. I know. I know. Just really limit it, OK? I've read that drinking a beer can be like eating five slices of bread. It's loaded with carbs, plus here too, the carbonation is very acidic. There's a reason that the typical, unsightly gut bulge is called a "beer belly." But my approach is not all-or-nothing. I still enjoy a beer every so often.

6. Avoid dairy. Initially, this idea was surprising to me, but over time, the majority of natural-health doctors and nutritionists I come across

recommend avoiding dairy. When you think about it, you realize that the amount of money the dairy industry spends on advertising and creating a healthy image is staggering. It's as if we've been brainwashed. Dairy's purpose in life is to turn a small animal into a large animal. When I look around, I see too many two-legged cows in our country. Unless you're trying to gain weight, or want more acne, constipation and inflammation in your body, I recommend avoiding dairy. Constipation is your body telling you that it does not know how to process something you ate. This is especially true if the milk has been pasteurized, which kills much of the food value, and homogenized, which restructures the milk. If you must have milk for some reason, many recommend switching to organic, raw whole milk. It is common in Europe, and studies have shown that it conveys health benefits when compared with processed milk, so do your own research on the validity of the common claims in the U.S. that raw milk is unsafe. Almond milk, especially organic, is a great substitute for dairy if you prefer to avoid it completely.

7. Limit carbs, including bread, pasta, grains and potatoes. Again, your body uses these carbs just like sugar. Rice or quinoa is a safer bet here, as some of you may have some sensitivity to the gluten in wheat, barley, rye, oats and other grains. A lot of people are gluten-sensitive. I sometimes have allergic reactions to bread and beer myself. Sometimes it's just a scratchy throat, or I may get a little wheezy.

8. Drink water with lemon. Mineral and spring water are best. Tap water quality depends on where you live, and you can always consider getting a good-quality water filter. If you drink out of a plastic bottle, you're drinking plastic chemicals. Glass is best. Stainless steel is next best. Water flushes toxins out of your system and keeps you regular. Do not underestimate the powerful health impact of simply switching to drinking water from other, unhealthier choices. The lemon juice contributes vitamin C, and it also turns into a powerful alkali (the opposite of acid) after digestion, which is very good for you.

9. Eat leafy greens. Organic greens usually aren't that much more expensive.

10. Eat more vegetables, excluding potatoes, preferably raw and organic if possible. Cooking or boiling vegetables can seriously deplete the amount of nutrients they contain. If you read a lot of natural health articles, over time you will learn that a lot of people have cured themselves from all sorts of health issues, simply by switching to a raw whole food diet.

11. Eat healthy fats, including:

    a. Avocados

    b. Olive oil

    c. Olives

    d. Nuts (my favorite snack)

    e. Eggs (add to salads or Asian food – the natural fat in the yolk will help boost fat-soluble vitamin absorption)

12. Eat organic meat, poultry and fish if you can afford it. The quality of regular meat, what the animals are fed and how they are treated, is really scary when you research it. For example, grass-fed beef is far superior to GMO-grain-fed beef. Cows were born to eat grass, so grass-fed cows are healthier. Some of my favorite meals now are salads with chicken or steak on top with an olive oil-based balsamic dressing. It's simple, nutritious and low on carbs. When I eat lunch at work I'm a huge Chipotle fan, as Chipotle's food is also GMO-free.

So the short recap is:

1. Avoid sugar.

2. Avoid table salt.

3. Avoid chemicals.

4. Avoid soda.

5. Avoid beer.

6. Avoid dairy.

7. Limit carbs, including bread, pasta, grains and potatoes.

8. Drink water with lemon. (This is the easiest, and it's huge for your health.)

9. Eat leafy greens, organic preferred.

10. Eat vegetables (excluding potatoes), raw and organic preferred.

11. Eat healthy fats: avocados, olive oil, olives, nuts, and eggs

12. Eat organic meat, poultry and fish

Why Eat More Healthy Fats?

There are two types of vitamins: water soluble and fat soluble. You need to eat fat to get, and be able to process, all those wonderful fat-soluble vitamins: A, D, E and K.

For years we were told to eat a low-fat, low-cholesterol diet. Did you know that the fattiest organ in your body is your brain? A New York Times Bestseller written by renowned neurologist David Perlmutter with contributions by Kristin Loberg, called *Grain Brain: The Surprising Truth about Wheat, Carbs, and Sugar – Your Brain's Silent Killers* explains that your brain requires fat and cholesterol to be healthy, and how carbs can actually damage your brain.

Think about the increase in Alzheimer's disease in our country. Looking at the Alzheimer's Association's home page, www.alz.org/facts, it says, "The number of Americans living with Alzheimer's disease is growing – and growing fast. An estimated 5.4 million

Americans of all ages have Alzheimer's disease in 2016... One in nine people age 65 and older has Alzheimer's disease... These numbers will escalate rapidly in coming years."

Could our low-fat, low-cholesterol diet be contributing to the increase in Alzheimer's? Researchers Perlmutter, Loberg and others say yes.

Here's another reason for aging men to consider eating more healthy fats: Did you know that testosterone is made from cholesterol?

How to Measure Success When You Change Eating Habits:

Very few people can just flip a switch and instantly change everything they've been eating. This is not an all-or-nothing proposition. Expect that it will take some time to adapt. I still eat some carbs. I still drink some beer. I still like an occasional slice of pie or scoop of ice cream.

I think Anthony Robbins is a genius. In his book *Awaken the Giant Within,* he explains that we have tied associations to a habit. For example, his first experience with alcohol was a terrible one that made him sick, so now, that association makes it easy for him to choose not to drink. People who choose to drink alcohol associate it with something positive, like relaxation or fun, and that is why they continue to drink. What is extremely powerful here is this: You can change your behavior simply by changing what you associate with that behavior.

Here's one of my own examples: When I learned that when I eat sugar, the first thing I feed is cancer cells, I immediately changed my association of sugar from something of pleasure to something much, much darker. I still eat the occasional sweet, but my consumption of sugar is down probably ninety percent or more. I am confident I will be able to limit my sugar intake for the rest of my days. This was an easy switch for me. My association between running and those line drills in high school basketball has been more difficult to change, but the good feelings I get from the Executive Workout™ is making it easier and easier for me to do sprints.

Think about the foods you like that you know are bad for you. We all have our weaknesses. What association have you made with that food? Sometimes these foods are associated with good memories and feelings. Think about what other habits you have in life. What association have you made with those habits? This is truly a deep concept depending on the extent you choose to explore it.

Pay attention to how you feel after eating something. Once I started eating healthy foods, it was easy to notice that my body did not feel good after eating fast food or junk food. After eating "clean" for the first three months, I was in a hurry one day and got some drive-through cheeseburgers. Soon afterward I felt so bad, so disgusting, I wanted to puke; but I was with clients. Good food is life giving, and you'll feel energized after eating it. Your body will tell you what is good and what is not. For unhealthy foods, I changed my association from the pleasure of eating the food to the not-so-great feeling – the opposite of pleasure – that I had after eating it.

So here's my suggestion to set you up for success. First, win the day. Then, if you can, win the week. For example, let's say on Tuesday you eat three meals. If at least two out of those three meals meet the above criteria, you win the day. Keep score each day. If you win at least four days out of the week, you win the week. Make sense?

If you focus on winning each day, you will win this battle, and before you realize it you will be feeling great, which will inspire you to win more meals, days and weeks. If you are achieving your goals, I encourage you to celebrate with a treat and not feel guilty. Again, this is not an all-or-nothing proposition. Live a little. Life is short. Enjoy the journey.

If Your Goal is to Lose Weight, Lose Fat or Increase Endurance:

The above plan will work great for you. It will turn you into a fat-burning inferno as you tap into your energy reserves. When I switched to this way of eating, my family was concerned for my health because the pounds had melted off my body so fast with very little exercise. So if losing weight and/or fat is your goal, when you look into your eyes in the mirror, tell yourself that you are a fat-burning inferno. Picture the new you, and visualize that you're achieving whatever goal is driving you.

One important tip. Always try to eat at least two to three hours before bedtime. This is better for digestion and sleep, and it will also burn off those carbs so that you can burn fat all night long. If you are still carb-fueled, this can be challenging from a hunger point of view, but once you're fat-fueled it shouldn't be an issue.

From a protein point of view, you shouldn't need to consume extra protein to lose weight.

If your Goal is to Build Muscle:

The above plan should be modified to greatly increase your protein intake while you're in the muscle-building phase. You also may need to eat more carbs. If you're following the ketogenic guidelines, it can be more difficult to maintain ketosis, as your body can also use protein as a fuel, instead of fat, and convert it to glucose. If you are following the workout routine in this book and you don't see gains in strength and muscle immediately in the first week or two, the most likely reason is that you are not eating enough. To build new muscle, you need to give the body lots of nutritious food and protein.

When I gained six and a half pounds of muscle in five weeks, here's what a typical day of eating looked like:

- Breakfast – As soon as I got up, I would make my favorite smoothie:
    - 1 Banana
    - Frozen organic blueberries ~ 1/3 cup
    - Frozen organic strawberries ~ 1/2 cup
    - Organic raw whole milk or almond milk
    - Chia seeds ~ 1 tablespoon
    - Whey protein powder ~ 1 scoop (18g of protein)
    - Organic raw apple cider vinegar ~ a generous splash .There are entire health books

dedicated to this amazing food. Make sure you include it.

- o Broccoli sprouts ~ these can dominate the flavor, so the amount is up to you. Kale or "power greens" are other popular options

- o If you don't enjoy fruit, many people use peanut butter or almond butter instead, and you might want to revisit adding the vinegar and sprouts.

- Mid-Morning Snack – Either two hard-boiled eggs, or nuts and a twenty-gram protein bar

- Lunch – Chipotle rice bowl, or salad with brown rice or beans, meat, salsa, guacamole and lettuce

- Mid-Afternoon Snack – Nuts and a twenty-gram protein bar

- Dinner – Organic meat or fish with organic veggies, for example:

  o Steak or chicken breast, potato or green beans, and salad or broccoli

  o Chicken fajitas – Chicken, caramelized onion and red pepper, salsa, guacamole and soft tortilla

  o Burger with a salad

  o Bourbon chicken and broccoli on rice

  o Fish and asparagus or other veggies

- Evening – If I worked out, I'd eat at least half a whey protein bar immediately before the workout unless it was too close to my bedtime food below. Whey protein is absorbed by the body quickly, so it's perfect for pre- or post-workout.

- Before Bedtime – Peanut butter or almond butter smoothie. Or, a quicker way to consume whey protein is to stir it into a short glass of freshly squeezed orange juice. It tastes like a creamsicle. Consider that orange juice is high in fructose (fruit sugar), though, so it may not mesh with your goals. If you're concerned about gaining fat weight, you can try skipping this or just have something smaller, like a hard-boiled egg or a handful of nuts. But if you're following the workout and not gaining strength and muscle quickly, don't skip this step.

About the above level of protein intake: There are potentially some health concerns about consuming so much protein for an extended period of time. I only recommend this level of protein in your diet if you're trying to build muscle quickly. Too much protein can impact something called the mTOR metabolic pathway, which may lead to increased cancer and other health risks.

Chapter 6

What's in Your Food?

As I've gotten older, raised my children and talked with other parents and people in general, a lot of things about food have become clear to me. I devour information on personal health. In talking with others, I find that most people have no idea how the body processes certain foods or what chemicals are in most of the food they are eating, and what those food types and chemicals might do to their own and their children's health.

Watch some documentaries on food, like *Food Inc.* – a 2008 American documentary directed by filmmaker Robert Krenner. Watch some Ted Talks about food at www.TED.com. There are also websites dedicated to natural health. One of my personal favorites is by Dr. Mercola at www.mercola.com. He also has a daily newsletter, which is a great way to keep abreast of new studies and events.

Did you know that chemicals are added to our food without necessarily being adequately tested? Or that the tests are provided solely by the chemical or food company whose profits depend on having that chemical pass the test? There is a strong correlation between favorable test results and funding by the interested party, which should not be a surprise.

There are much more stringent requirements in Europe, where chemicals have to undergo more-rigorous testing before being added to food. Especially in the U.S., you should consider educating yourself about what's in your food. If something is not approved in Europe for human consumption, that should at least be a red flag for you that it's something worth researching further.

Consider paying more attention to what you and your family eat, and what happens afterward. Below are some examples of the most important things I've learned about food over the last several years. My goal is simply to show you the biggest issues to be aware of, and then, I hope, to motivate you to take an interest in food. It's a simple, yet powerful way to improve your own health, and the health of your loved ones. This first issue is the most important issue by far.

GMO (Genetically Modified Organisms):

Most people I talk to about food don't know what "GMO" means. The Chipotle restaurant chain advertises that its menu is "GMO free." There is an epic battle going on regarding GMOs between chemical companies like Monsanto and governments here and abroad. Some states are trying to pass labeling laws that would require food companies to label products that contain GMOs. In October 2015, nineteen European countries, including France and Germany – more than half the countries in the European Union, in fact – banned GMO crops. Dozens of other countries have banned them as well. Why?

Google "GMO foods" or "GMO cereal." I just Googled "Does Europe allow GMO foods?" and came across some fascinating articles. I find that foreign media is often more open, and less biased towards big business, than our media in the U.S.

GMO crops, which were first approved in 1996, are prevalent in the U.S. More than ninety percent of all corn and soybean acreage in the U.S. is already GMO. Sugar beets are another prominent GMO crop. GMO crops have had their DNA altered with genes from completely different organisms. But perhaps more of an issue is that these crops are usually treated with a chemical pesticide called glyphosate, which the World Health Organization (WHO) has classified as a "probable human carcinogen." Other scientists also allege that this chemical causes all kinds of other health effects.

As I write this in December, 2016, California is trying to add glyphosate to its list of known carcinogens, but Monsanto, the manufacturer of the weed-killer Roundup, which contains glyphosate, is suing California in attempt to stop glyphosate from being put on the known carcinogen list. In its fiscal year 2015,

Monsanto generated $4.8 billion in revenue from sales of Roundup. I wonder how many legal challenges and scientific studies are being fought by Monsanto all around the world.

Stop and think about how pervasive an issue this is. Corn is an ingredient in a huge variety of foods, and it comes in literally hundreds of different forms – including corn oil, vegetable oil, corn syrup, high-fructose corn syrup, corn meal, corn starch, cellulose, ascorbic acid, citric acid, dextrose and many more. Soy is similarly pervasive. Corn and soybean oil are everywhere, so if you're eating out and getting fried food or salad dressing, it likely contains GMO oil. Most sugar in the U.S. comes from sugar beets, not sugar cane.

The safest way to avoid these GMO products and associated chemicals is to buy and eat organic food, or find places to eat that are GMO free.

Why Eat Organic?

There are a few hugely important reasons why you should consider eating organic food:

- To avoid GMOs and associated chemicals.
- According to a Mayo Clinic article at www.mayoclinic.org, written by Mayo Clinic Staff, entitled "Organic foods: Are they safer? More nutritious?":
  - "Organic produce typically carries significantly fewer pesticide residues than does conventional produce."
  - "Organic regulations ban or severely restrict the use of food additives, processing aids

(substances used during processing, but not added directly to food) and fortifying agents commonly used in nonorganic foods, including preservatives, artificial sweeteners, colorings and flavorings, and monosodium glutamate (MSG)."

o "Organic farming practices are designed to benefit the environment by reducing pollution and conserving water and soil quality."

Aspartame

Aspartame is an artificial sweetener that's sold under the Nutrasweet and Equal brands. It is two hundred times sweeter than sugar, so companies save a lot of money by only using a little aspartame instead of two hundred times more sugar.

It is a common ingredient in:

- diet soda

- chewing gum

- pudding

- gelatin

- lemonade

- iced tea

- hot chocolate

- other sweetened products.

Aspartame got into our food supply in 1981. In 1995, the FDA reported that aspartame complaints were responsible for more complaints than all others combined for that fourteen-year period. There is a long list of potential side effects, including:

- vision impairment

- headaches

- migraines

- memory loss

- vomiting or nausea

- abdominal pain and cramps

- diarrhea

- weight gain

- heart palpitation

- severe depression or anxiety attacks

- and many others. Google "FDA aspartame side effects."

I know multiple people who had migraines, and after they gave up diet soda, their migraines went away.

One article I read said that there was an overwhelming tendency for both industry-funded and FDA-funded studies to say that aspartame is okay, but the overwhelming majority of privately funded studies found at least one issue with aspartame. This is why you have to educate yourself. Whenever you see results published from a research study, you need to find out who funded the study. The chemical companies fund their own studies, and the media reports those results to you. Do you understand?

Educate yourself. Open your eyes and ears. Much of what you hear in the media is what the companies whose profits are at stake want you to hear. They care more about their profits than about your and your family's health. You will see it with your own eyes, if you don't already. People are getting sicker at earlier ages. Maybe, just maybe, it has something to do with what's in our food.

Trans Fat from Partially Hydrogenated Oils:

According to www.fda.gov, "...eating trans fat raises the level of low-density lipoprotein (LDL or "bad") cholesterol in the blood. An elevated LDL blood cholesterol level can increase your risk of developing cardiovascular disease. Cardiovascular disease is the leading cause of death in both men and women in the U.S. Therefore, you should keep your intake of trans fat as low as possible."

The FDA has released its final determination that Partially Hydrogenated Oils (PHOs) are not Generally Recognized as Safe (GRAS). In the release, it says, "Removing PHOs from processed foods could prevent thousands of heart attacks and deaths each year." If you ask me, this is nasty stuff.

Trans fats are formed when hydrogen is added to vegetable oil to make it more solid. Food manufacturers use them to improve the texture, shelf life and flavor stability of foods.

Food companies have two options. One, they must work to remove trans fats from food. Or two, they must petition the FDA for permission to use PHOs. On my last trip to the grocery store (December 2016), I looked through the ingredients list of multiple brands of crackers, plus muffin and pancake mixes – and partially hydrogenated oils were still listed in nearly all the products. Avoid partially hydrogenated oils!

Common foods that contain partially hydrogenated oils (trans fat) are:

- Vegetable shortenings and stick margarines

- Coffee creamer

- Crackers, cookies, cakes, muffins, pancakes, frozen pies & other baked goods

- Fast food

- Frozen pizza

- Ready-to-use frostings

- Refrigerated dough products (i.e. biscuits, cinnamon rolls)

- Snack foods like microwave popcorn

Aluminum:

Many articles have been written about the potentially harmful health effects of aluminum. Aluminum goes straight to your brain, and it is hard to get out of your body, so it accumulates. Some studies have indicated a possible link to neurological diseases such as Alzheimer's. As with many of these issues, there are ongoing debates, with industry funding behind one side. To be safe, my recommendation is to avoid aluminum.

Aluminum is prevalent in a great many products, and food is sometimes cooked or stored in aluminum. Look for it in these products – for many of these, there are

alternatives that are aluminum-free:

- Baking powder

- Salt

- Baby formula

- Coffee creamers

- Baked goods

- Drugs like antacids

- Deodorants

- Cosmetics

- Shampoo

- Toothpaste

- Vaccines

- Aluminum cans, foil, juice pouches, food trays

- Aluminum cookware

Learn How Foods Are Processed (Examples – Orange Juice and Milk):

One thing about my oldest daughter Tatum: she loves oranges. She used to eat as many as four or five oranges per day when orange season first came into full swing. I struggled to keep them stocked in the refrigerator. One day I asked her if she wanted orange juice from the grocery store. She said, "No thanks. I don't like orange juice." It seems so funny to me now, but I had never thought about it until that moment. Does the orange juice you buy at the store taste like oranges? No is the answer, unless it's truly fresh-squeezed.

Alissa Hamilton wrote a book called *Squeezed: What You Don't Know About Orange Juice*. I had always thought that "juice not from concentrate" was a good, healthy thing. The truth is, however, that the juice companies can store orange juice for months in tanks. Since fresh juice only lasts two or three days, in order to store it longer they remove the oxygen from the juice, which destroys its natural flavors. They also have to pasteurize the juice to kill any bacteria that have grown after all this time in storage. Later, the juice companies add chemical flavor packs to give the juice its orange-like flavor and aroma. This is why each brand always has a consistent flavor, and why each brand's flavor is different from the others, even though the original oranges may have come from the same source.

The result is that now we get to enjoy this unhealthy industrial product all year long. Is it still juice? Is it food? I guess that depends on how you define food.

Have you ever had a chance to drink fresh raw milk?

It's quite different from the milk you buy in the store.

Grocery-store milk is highly processed. Usually it is

pasteurized and homogenized so that it lasts much

longer and the cream doesn't separate, boosting the

milk companies' profits. Any time a food is modified

so that it lasts much longer, I am skeptical that my body

will still process it like a natural food. As I've

mentioned, constipation is a sign that your body

doesn't know how to process something you've eaten.

"Pasteurized" milk can last for two to three weeks,

while "ultra-pasteurized" milk can last up to nine

months!

When my oldest teenage daughter, Tatum, cut out

dairy, not only did her allergies disappear, 100%, but

her acne also cleared up significantly. There are a lot

of people who have had similar experiences. To see if dairy is affecting your health, just give it up for one week and see if you notice any changes.

The only time I might recommend keeping dairy in your diet is if your goal is to bulk up, and you've been struggling to get there without dairy. Drinking a lot of milk is a great way to help you bulk up.

Quick Recap:

1. Avoid Genetically Modified Organism (GMO) foods

2. Eat organic as much as possible

3. Avoid aspartame

4. Avoid trans fats from Partially Hydrogenated Oils (PHOs)

5. Avoid aluminum

6. Learn how foods are processed, for example, orange juice and dairy

Chapter 7

Other Vital Health Tips

This chapter is dedicated to the other things you may want to consider for living a healthier life. Again, I'm giving you just the "big rocks" (as Stephen Covey puts it) that will give you the most benefit.

Sitting is the New Smoking:

Dr. James Levine – director of the Mayo Clinic-Arizona State University Obesity Solutions Initiative, and inventor of the treadmill desk – is credited with coining the phrase, "Sitting is the new smoking." Mounting evidence continues to show that prolonged sitting has several serious health consequences, including increased risk for various types of cancer, type 2 diabetes and heart disease – and it obviously isn't good for our backs, either.

In a Los Angeles Times article by Mary MacVean entitled "'Get Up!' Or lose hours of your life every day, scientist says," Dr. Levine is quoted as saying, "Sitting is more dangerous than smoking, kills more people than HIV and is more treacherous than parachuting. We are sitting ourselves to death." Further, he writes, "We lose two hours of life for every hour we sit."

What is key to understand here is this: the effects of sitting are not reversible through exercise or other healthy habits. Your only option here is to reduce the amount of time you spend on your rear end. I have a standing desk at home that I use fairly often. As much as possible, try not to sit for more than twenty minutes at a time. Set a timer. Get up and move around regularly throughout the day. Life is motion.

Gut Bacteria and Probiotics:

"All disease begins in the gut." – Hippocrates

There is a growing body of scientific evidence that illustrates how important your gut bacteria are to your health. If you can't properly digest the food you eat, what you eat won't matter much. You have "good bacteria" in your digestive system that help you process food. Some studies have shown that adding "probiotics" (good bacteria contained in foods or supplements) to your diet may boost your immune system. When you take antibiotics, you kill both the good and bad bacteria in your body. Processed foods and other ingested chemicals are not kind to your good bacteria either.

So eat clean to keep your gut bacteria healthy. Probiotics such as fermented foods (including pickles and sauerkraut), organic apple-cider vinegar, yogurt and kombucha can help your body replenish these good bacteria. You should consult a physician about taking probiotics, particularly if you have an impaired immune system.

Vitamin D:

There are so many purported benefits of vitamin D, it's the closest thing I've found to a silver bullet for good health. It's also inexpensive. Judging by study results, the estimates of how many people in the U.S. are vitamin D deficient vary widely, but the consensus is that it's a huge issue. On the high end, as much as seventy-five percent of the population could be vitamin D deficient, according to a March 23, 2009 article in Scientific American entitled "Vitamin D deficiency soars in the U.S., study says." The deficiency numbers are even higher for darker-skinned populations like blacks and Hispanics.

Vitamin D has many functions in your body, and mounting evidence suggests that vitamin D deficiency could be linked to osteoporosis, depression, high blood pressure, and many chronic conditions, including cardiovascular disease, multiple sclerosis, type 1 diabetes and several cancers. It plays a vital role in cellular functions and it is important to your immune system. Vitamin D, in fact, is involved in the function of ALL cells and tissues in your body.

In a webmd.com archives article entitled "Vitamin D: Vital Role in Your Health," author Michael F. Holick, PhD, MD, who heads the Vitamin D, Skin, and Bone

Research Laboratory at Boston University School of Medicine, writes, "Activated vitamin D is one of the most potent inhibitors of cancer cell growth. It also stimulates your pancreas to make insulin. It regulates your immune system."

Your body produces vitamin D naturally from sunlight, but this varies greatly, based on your proximity to the equator, and therefore, how direct the sunlight is. In winter months, your body produces minimal, if any, vitamin D from sunlight.

Think about how crucial sunlight is for photosynthesis in plants. In my view, sunlight is likely just as important for the human body, as your skin is made to synthesize sunlight into vitamin D. I believe adequate sunlight and vitamin D are both crucial for good health.

We were not made to be cave trolls. Get some sun on your skin. Obviously, though, don't overdo it.

If it's a time of year where the days are shorter and the sun is lower in the sky, I highly recommend supplementing with vitamin D3, specifically, not any other type of vitamin D supplement. It's really inexpensive, and I take it most days between summers. I believe that this is one of the keys to why my immune system has been bulletproof over the last seven years.

Cleansing:

In Chapter 5, Number 3 on my "what to eat and what not to eat" list is "Avoid chemicals." So, if you're diligent, you will greatly reduce the amount of chemicals coming into your body. The next important step is to get rid of the chemicals that are already being stored in your body. These can cause a toxic overload, which can potentially interfere with any of the body's chemical-sensitive processes. If you don't think you store toxins in your body, have you ever gotten a massage?

The masseur or masseuse always tells you to drink a lot of water afterward, to help flush out the stored toxins from your system that the massage has released. Some people even feel sick after a massage, because so much toxic material gets released that it temporarily overwhelms their system. When a person sweats, if it smells bad, that can be an indication of toxins in his system. A cleansed person will sweat a normal, salty scent.

If you read a lot of natural health articles the way I do, you will see many cases where people have cured different ailments simply by driving toxins out of their

117

system and eating clean food. For me, cleansing is absolutely vital to good health.

There are a lot of ways to cleanse. My favorites are:

1. Always drink at least 20 ounces of water with lemon after you get up in the morning. Mineral or spring water is best. This helps to keep you regular and flush you out. If you're not regular, the toxins in your waste go into your bloodstream – so get them out!

2. Take a hot bath with one cup of baking soda, two cups of Epsom salts, and ten drops of lavender essential oil. Drink a lot of water with lemon during and afterward. Such heat can be dangerous if you have certain health conditions, like cardiovascular issues, so consult a doctor. The sudden change from cold

to hot can cause heart attacks. If you're weak from an illness, it increases the risk of you fainting. Take a hot bath with a partner if you can. Be careful.

3. Take a sauna. Sweating in a sauna is a great way to get toxins out. A far-infrared sauna is even better, as it heats your tissues several inches deep. Drink a lot of water with lemon during and afterward. Consult a doctor to make sure a sauna is safe for you, and be aware of the similar possible issues mentioned above with the hot bath.

4. Have a massage, followed by lemon water.

5. Try fasting. Have you ever noticed that when a pet is sick, its instinct is not to eat? Fasting gives your digestive organs a chance to rest, and it is very cleansing. Some scientists

believe that fasting triggers your stem cells to release their powerful healing forces. Ancient Greeks used fasting to treat everything from the common cold to severe illnesses. You can simply stick to water for a day, or a low-calorie liquid, like juice. Many people, in fact, recommend doing a juice cleanse for up to three days. a) Intermittent Fasting – You go for up to fifteen or sixteen hours out of twenty-four without eating solid food. The easiest way is to eat an early dinner and then not eat again until fifteen hours later the following day. So if you had dinner at 6 PM, you wouldn't eat solid food again until at least 9 AM. This gives you many of the same benefits as a hard-core traditional fast, and you're essentially fasting while you're sleeping, so it's much easier.

6. There are many different cleanses you can take orally, including supplement-type capsules. I've done a couple of these, but I don't want to recommend anything.

I Like It Hot:

"Give me a fever and I can cure any disease."

Hippocrates

It's not a coincidence that two of my favorite cleanse methods, hot bath and sauna, involve heat. Your body naturally uses heat from a fever to destroy invaders. As it turns out, viruses and bad bacteria tend to have weaker cell walls, so they are much more susceptible to being destroyed by heat than regular cells are.

Again, a far-infrared sauna heats your tissues several inches deep, so I am a huge fan. Additionally, the heat increases both blood flow and oxygenation to your tissues, which are also bad for invaders – and good for reducing inflammation and general healing.

Stress – The Silent Killer:

We know that stress is an unavoidable factor in our lives, and that it can have serious impacts on our health over both the short and the long term. An online article called "Stress symptoms: Effects on your body and behavior," by Mayo Clinic Staff on www.mayoclinic.org, says, "You may think illness is to blame for that nagging headache, your frequent insomnia or your decreased productivity at work. But stress may actually be the culprit. Stress that's left unchecked can contribute to many health problems, such as high blood pressure, heart disease, obesity and diabetes."

Anxiety, depression, irritability, overeating, skipping meals, a weakened immune system, headaches, and fatigue are common signs of stress. Find healthy things that relax you, and do them regularly. Listening to music, exercising, reading or vegging out to a movie or TV are the most common methods. I'm also a big fan of meditation and yoga. Get outside and connect with nature. If you do a hot bath, sauna or massage, you're killing two birds with one stone: getting some healthy cleansing while you relax. It's also important to disconnect from work and take vacations.

Krill Oil:

Krill oil is my second-favorite supplement, after vitamin D3. A lot of people take fish oil. Krill oil, extracted from tiny, shrimp-like crustaceans, is loaded with omega-3 fatty acids and the powerful antioxidant, astaxanthin. It is superior to fish oil because it comes from a sustainable source, avoids the fishy taste and, unlike fish, contains little or no mercury. The benefits of krill oil include:

- Upholds brain health, learning and memory
- Supports cardiovascular health
- Helps maintain healthy cholesterol and blood-sugar levels
- Reduces inflammation
- Boosts immune function
- Improves joint function
- Is good for your skin

The research and benefits documented for krill oil are outstanding.

Watch What You Put on Your Skin:

When you put a liquid or other product on your skin, your skin absorbs it. Unlike your digestive system when you eat something, your skin does not have any filters. So, just as you read labels for the food you eat, you need to read labels for the products you're putting on your skin. You will find that deodorants, lotions, cosmetics, soaps, shampoos and other things are loaded with unhealthy chemicals.

The good news is that there are healthier options you can find online at websites for natural foods and products, or at retailers like Whole Foods, Trader Joe's, Sprouts and more.

Grounding or Earthing

I briefly mentioned earlier that we are like alkaline batteries, continuously producing heat and energy. Just like an electrical outlet, we need to be grounded. In this electronic age, our bodies constantly build up positive charges, or free radicals, via Wi-Fi, cellular, hi-def devices, and more. Simply coming into contact with the earth grounds us, and our buildup of positive electrons transfers to the earth as we pick up negatively charged free electrons, which is a good thing. Your electrical charge becomes the same as the earth's.

Earthing has many potential benefits, including:

- Better sleep
- Stress reduction
- Inflammation reduction
- Pain reduction

- Increased energy

- Improved blood pressure and circulation

- Improved healing ability

Many of you probably enjoy nature already, so now you have a little science to explain one of the reasons why it's so healthy. So take some time to enjoy and connect with mother earth. Walk barefoot, sit on the ground or on a rock or tree stump. Get your hands dirty and plant a garden. In the summer months, I often play on my back lawn with the dogs for fifteen minutes with just shorts on, so I get my healthy sunlight and earthing at the same time. Simply switching from rubber-soled shoes to leather will help you connect better. There are even devices you can use indoors, such as earthing sheets for your bed, so that you become grounded while you sleep.

Quick Recap

1. Sitting is the new smoking

2. Take care of your gut bacteria

3. Vitamin D, get some summer sun on your skin or supplement with vitamin D3

4. Cleansing

   a) Drink a lot of water with lemon, preferably mineral or spring water

   b) Hot baths

   c) Sauna

   d) Massage

   e) Fasting or intermittent fasting

5. Krill oil supplements

6. Watch what you put on your skin

7.   Ground or earth yourself

Chapter 8

Corporate Wellness for Employers

Your employees may spend more time at work than they do with their loved ones. Make their work environment a healthy one, and both you and they will benefit from their improved health in many different ways. Increased job satisfaction, better attendance, higher employee retention, enhanced productivity and heightened creativity are just a few of these.

Here's what you can do to help bring this about:

1. Educate your employees by offering them this book, and/or other health and nutrition classes and materials.

2. Offer organic, non-GMO and chemical-free foods and snacks onsite. One of my best friends works for Intel, and they have local farmers come in and sell organic produce onsite at specific times during the week.

3. Offer employees standing desks or exercise balls to sit on.

4. Create lunch, meeting and social areas where people can stand or walk around, both inside and outdoors. If you need to talk with someone, have a "walk-n-talk." If it's a nice day, take it outside.

5. Encourage employees to use timers, so that they stand up and move a little every twenty minutes.

6. Make the work environment a little more like home. Bring in more natural light or, if that's not an option, switch to light bulbs that are closer to natural light instead of dim fluorescent bulbs. Put in windows or ventilation systems that bring in fresh air. And for crying out loud, bring some life to the place. Put some color on the walls – and get away from gray, tan or brown. Add art and other bright touches. And put some real plants around the office for their beauty and natural feel – as well as the oxygen they provide.

7. Create attractive and relaxing areas outside for employees to escape momentarily and enjoy the invigorating outdoor fresh air.

8. Put a gym in your building. The Executive Workout™ only takes ten to fifteen minutes. People could schedule the room for fifteen-minute sessions, as they would a conference room. At least offer to pay for gym memberships.

9. Offer yoga or other classes onsite. These can be before, after or during work hours.

10. All of the above ideas are opportunities to show your employees that you care about them. Show you care, then involve and empower them in the above initiatives. This is a true win-win.

Chapter 9

Wrap-up

I hope that you've found some things in this book that will improve your and your loved ones' health, happiness and quality of life. If you have not been paying attention to what's in your food, I hope that this book has increased your awareness of why it may be critical to your health. If you want to dive deeper, there are entire books dedicated to each topic touched upon in this book.

With just one hour of exercise per week, as described in the Executive Workout™, eating the right foods, avoiding chemicals and following a few additional healthy habits, I believe that most people will feel

tremendously better, look better, have more energy —
and live longer, happier, more fulfilled lives.

I am grateful to you for taking the time to read this
book. Thank you.